YOU CAN

END OF STORY.

HEALTH & WELLNESS

Big Goals
Give your Goals a Date
Give your Goals a Plan
Before & After Photos
Measurement Tracker
Goal Tracker
Weight Loss Tracker

Nutrition for 90 Days

Weekly Meal Planner
Grocery List
Daily Food Journal

Fitness for 90 Days

Monthly Workout Planner
Monthly Cardio Tracker
Weekly Strength Training Tracker

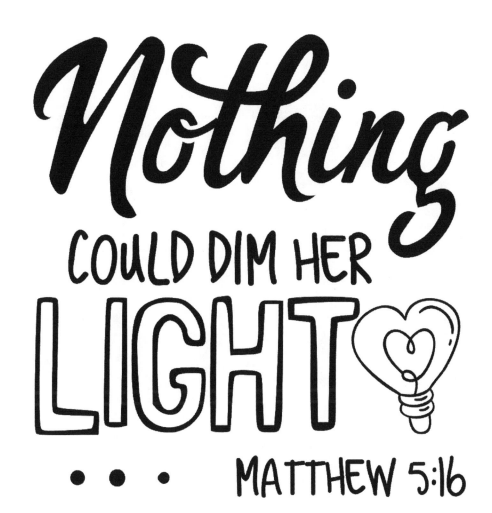

Nothing COULD DIM HER LIGHT

MATTHEW 5:16

General Health Goals

Goal # 1

Goal # 2

Goal # 3

Goal # 4

General Health Goals

Goal # 5

Goal # 6

Goal # 7

Goal # 8

ACTION PLAN FOR WELLNESS GOALS

Goal		Date

My Progress

Motivation	My Why	Truth statements

Habits	Habits to Start	Habits to stop

Support	accountability plan	partner(s)

Nutrition Plan	focus	meal/snack schedule

plenty of	some of	limit/avoid

Daily Nutrition Goals

calories	fat	carbs	protein	fiber	sugar

Fitness Plan	physical activity	strength training

physical activity	strength training

Lifestyle Plan — Lifestyle plan for continued wellness

celebrate		date

ACTION PLAN FOR WEIGHT LOSS GOAL

Goal		Date

My Progress

Motivation

My Why	Truth Statement

Habits

Habits to Start	Habits to stop

Support

accountability plan	partner(s)

FOCUS	MEAL/SNACK SCHEDULE

Nutrition Plan

PLENTY OF	SOME OF	LIMIT/AVOID

Daily Nutrition Goals

calories	fat	carbs	protein	fiber	sugar

Fitness Plan

Physical Activity	Strength Training

Lifestyle Plan

Weight Maintenance Plan

Celebrate		Date

My Action Plan for Fitness Goal

Goal		Date

My Progress

Motivation	My Why	Truth Statement

Goal Progress & Details	Schedule	Healthy Habits	Benchmarks to meet
	Starting Stats		
	Final Stats		

Support	Accountability Plan

Celebrate		Date

MY BEFORE & AFTER PHOTOS

Before

Picture Here

After

Picture Here

MY HEALTH STATS

• • • • • • • • • • Goal Time Frame • • • • • • • • • •

3 months _____

Health Indicator	Starting	Goal	Final	+/-
Blood Pressure				
Weight				
Endurance				
Strength				
Confidence				

My Weekly Measurements

Things to Measure	Date		Date		Date		Date	
	#	+/-	#	+/-	#	+/-	#	+/-
weight								
hips								
waist								
bust								
thigh								
neck								
bicep								

Things to Measure	Date		Date		Date		Date	
	#	+/-	#	+/-	#	+/-	#	+/-
weight								
hips								
waist								
bust								
thigh								
neck								
bicep								

My Weekly Measurements

Things to Measure	Date		Date		Date		Date	
	#	+/-	#	+/-	#	+/-	#	+/-
weight								
hips								
waist								
bust								
thigh								
neck								
bicep								

Things to Measure	Date		Date		Date		Date	
	#	+/-	#	+/-	#	+/-	#	+/-
weight								
hips								
waist								
bust								
thigh								
neck								
bicep								

PROGRESS TRACKER

Date	Goal	Actual	+/-	Next Steps

THIS IS THE YEAR
i will be
STRONGER
BRAVER
KINDER &
UNSTOPPABLE.
this year i will be
FIERCE.

The Meal Planner

Week One:

	BREAKFAST	LUNCH	DINNER	SNACKS
MON				
TUE				
WED				
THU				
FRI				
SAT				
SUN				

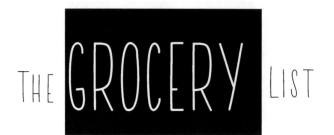

THE GROCERY LIST

Week One:_____

DAILY JOURNAL

Date

Food Journal

B

L

D

S

Habit Tracker

☆

☆

☆

☆

☆

☆

☆

Water Intake
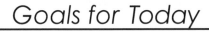

Weight

Workout: Cardio Strength or Rest

Goals for Today

Gratitude Statement

Sleep the Night Before

Celebrations & Struggles

DAILY JOURNAL

Date: _____

Food Journal

B

L

D

S

Habit Tracker

☆
☆
☆
☆
☆
☆
☆

Water Intake

Weight

Workout: Cardio Strength or Rest

Goals for Today

Gratitude Statement

Sleep the Night Before

Celebrations &Struggles

DAILY JOURNAL

Date:

Food Journal

B

L

D

S

Habit Tracker

☆

☆

☆

☆

☆

☆

☆

Water Intake

Weight

Workout: Cardio Strength or Rest

Goals for Today

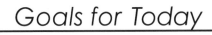

Gratitude Statement

Sleep the Night Before

Celebrations & Struggles

DAILY JOURNAL

Date: _____

Food Journal

B

L

D

S

Habit Tracker

☆
☆
☆
☆
☆
☆
☆

Water Intake

• Weight

Workout: Cardio Strength or Rest

Goals for Today

Gratitude Statement

Sleep the Night Before

Celebrations & Struggles

DAILY JOURNAL

Date _____

Food Journal

B

L

D

S

Habit Tracker

☆
☆
☆
☆
☆
☆
☆

Water Intake

Weight

Workout: Cardio Strength or Rest

Goals for Today

Gratitude Statement

Sleep the Night Before

Celebrations &Struggles

DAILY JOURNAL

Date: _____

Food Journal

B

L

D

S

Habit Tracker

☆

☆

☆

☆

☆

☆

☆

Water Intake

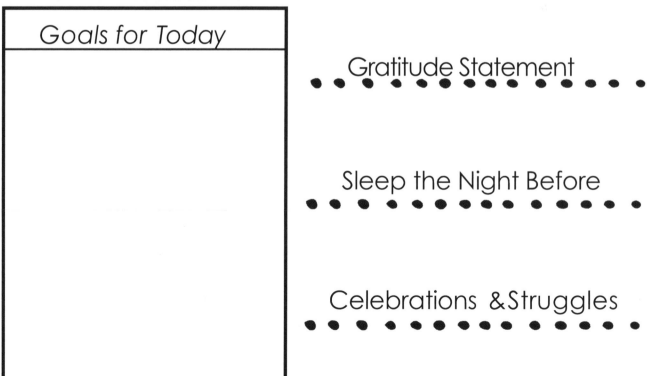

Weight

Workout: Cardio Strength or Rest

Goals for Today

Gratitude Statement

. . . .

Sleep the Night Before

. . . .

Celebrations & Struggles

. . . .

DAILY JOURNAL

Date:

Food Journal

B

L

D

S

Habit Tracker

☆

☆

☆

☆

☆

☆

☆

Water Intake

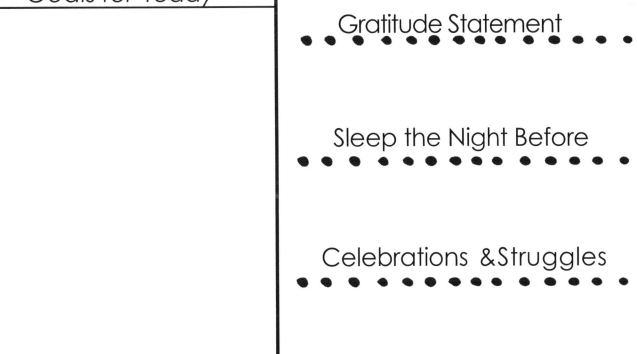

Weight

Workout: Cardio Strength or Rest

Goals for Today

Gratitude Statement

Sleep the Night Before

Celebrations &Struggles

The Meal Planner

	BREAKFAST	LUNCH	DINNER	SNACKS
MON				
TUE				
WED				
THU				
FRI				
SAT				
SUN				

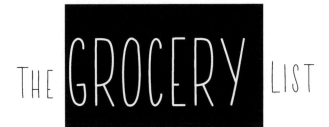

The GROCERY List

Week Two:_____

DAILY JOURNAL

Date:_____

Food Journal

B

L

D

S

Habit Tracker

☆
☆
☆
☆
☆
☆
☆

Water Intake

Weight

Workout: Cardio Strength or Rest

Goals for Today

Gratitude Statement

Sleep the Night Before

Celebrations &Struggles

DAILY JOURNAL

Date:

Food Journal

B

L

D

S

Habit Tracker

☆

☆

☆

☆

☆

☆

☆

Water Intake

Weight

Workout: Cardio Strength or Rest

Goals for Today

Gratitude Statement

Sleep the Night Before

Celebrations &Struggles

DAILY JOURNAL

Date: _____

Food Journal

B

L

D

S

Habit Tracker

☆
☆
☆
☆
☆
☆
☆

Water Intake

Weight

Workout: Cardio Strength or Rest

Goals for Today

Gratitude Statement

Sleep the Night Before

Celebrations & Struggles

DAILY JOURNAL

Date_____

Food Journal

B

L

D

S

Habit Tracker

☆
☆
☆
☆
☆
☆
☆

Water Intake

Weight

Workout: Cardio Strength or Rest

Goals for Today

Gratitude Statement

Sleep the Night Before

Celebrations & Struggles

DAILY JOURNAL

Date:_____

Food Journal

B

L

D

S

Habit Tracker

☆

☆

☆

☆

☆

☆

☆

Water Intake

Weight

Workout: Cardio Strength or Rest

Goals for Today

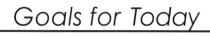

Gratitude Statement

Sleep the Night Before

Celebrations & Struggles

DAILY JOURNAL

Date:

Food Journal

B

L

D

S

Habit Tracker

☆

☆

☆

☆

☆

☆

☆

Water Intake

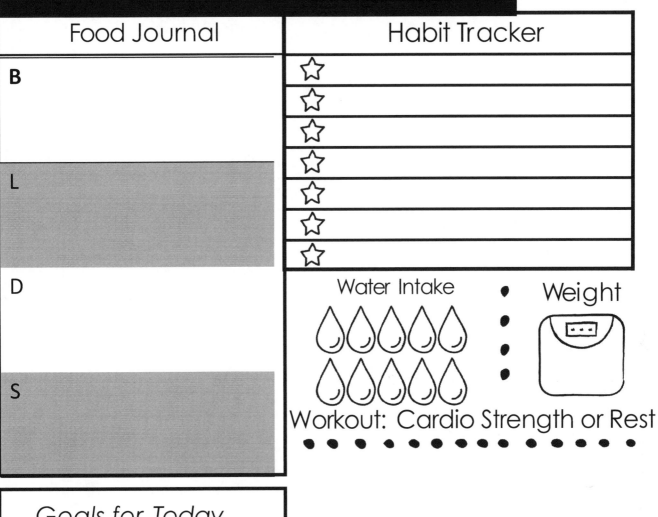

Weight

Workout: Cardio Strength or Rest

• • • • • • • • • • • • • • •

Goals for Today

Gratitude Statement

• • • • • • • • • • • • •

Sleep the Night Before

• • • • • • • • • • • • •

Celebrations & Struggles

• • • • • • • • • • • • •

DAILY JOURNAL

Date:_____

Food Journal

B

L

D

S

Habit Tracker

☆

☆

☆

☆

☆

☆

☆

Water Intake

Weight

Workout: Cardio Strength or Rest

Goals for Today

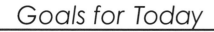

Gratitude Statement

Sleep the Night Before

Celebrations & Struggles

The Meal Planner

	BREAKFAST	LUNCH	DINNER	SNACKS
MON				
TUE				
WED				
THU				
FRI				
SAT				
SUN				

The GROCERY List

DAILY JOURNAL

Date

Food Journal

B

L

D

S

Habit Tracker

☆

☆

☆

☆

☆

☆

☆

Water Intake

Weight

Workout: Cardio Strength or Rest

• • • • • • • • • • • • • • • •

Goals for Today

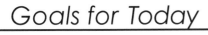

Gratitude Statement

• • • • • • • • • • • • • • •

Sleep the Night Before

• • • • • • • • • • • • • • •

Celebrations & Struggles

• • • • • • • • • • • • • • • •

DAILY JOURNAL

Date:_____

Food Journal

B

L

D

S

Habit Tracker

☆

☆

☆

☆

☆

☆

☆

Water Intake

Weight

Workout: Cardio Strength or Rest

Goals for Today

Gratitude Statement

Sleep the Night Before

Celebrations & Struggles

DAILY JOURNAL

Date: _____

Food Journal

B

L

D

S

Habit Tracker

☆

☆

☆

☆

☆

☆

☆

Water Intake

Weight

Workout: Cardio Strength or Rest

• • • • • • • • • • • • • • •

Goals for Today

Gratitude Statement

• • • • • • • • • • • • • •

Sleep the Night Before

• • • • • • • • • • • • • •

Celebrations & Struggles

• • • • • • • • • • • • • • •

DAILY JOURNAL

Date:_____

Food Journal

B

L

D

S

Habit Tracker

☆

☆

☆

☆

☆

☆

☆

Water Intake

Weight

Workout: Cardio Strength or Rest

Goals for Today

Gratitude Statement

Sleep the Night Before

Celebrations &Struggles

DAILY JOURNAL

Date:

Food Journal

B

L

D

S

Habit Tracker

☆

☆

☆

☆

☆

☆

☆

Water Intake

Weight

Workout: Cardio Strength or Rest
• • • • • • • • • • • • • •

Goals for Today

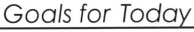

Gratitude Statement
• • • • • • • • • • • • •

Sleep the Night Before
• • • • • • • • • • • • • •

Celebrations &Struggles
• • • • • • • • • • • • • •

DAILY JOURNAL

Date: _____

Food Journal

B

L

D

S

Habit Tracker

☆
☆
☆
☆
☆
☆
☆

Water Intake

Weight

Workout: Cardio Strength or Rest

Goals for Today

Gratitude Statement

Sleep the Night Before

Celebrations & Struggles

DAILY JOURNAL

Date:

Food Journal

B

L

D

S

Habit Tracker

☆

☆

☆

☆

☆

☆

☆

Water Intake

Weight

Workout: Cardio Strength or Rest

Goals for Today

Gratitude Statement

Sleep the Night Before

Celebrations &Struggles

The Meal Planner

	BREAKFAST	LUNCH	DINNER	SNACKS
MON				
TUE				
WED				
THU				
FRI				
SAT				
SUN				

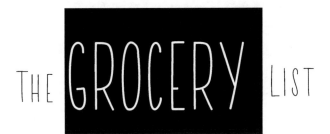

THE GROCERY LIST

Week Four:_____

DAILY JOURNAL

Date:_____

Food Journal

B

L

D

S

Habit Tracker

☆

☆

☆

☆

☆

☆

☆

Water Intake

Weight

Workout: Cardio Strength or Rest

Goals for Today

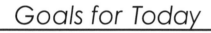

Gratitude Statement

Sleep the Night Before

Celebrations & Struggles

DAILY JOURNAL

Date: _____

Food Journal

B

L

D

S

Habit Tracker

☆

☆

☆

☆

☆

☆

☆

Water Intake

Weight

Workout: Cardio Strength or Rest

Goals for Today

Gratitude Statement

Sleep the Night Before

Celebrations &Struggles

DAILY JOURNAL

Date: _____

Food Journal

B

L

D

S

Habit Tracker

☆

☆

☆

☆

☆

☆

☆

Water Intake

Weight

Workout: Cardio Strength or Rest

• • • • • • • • • • • • •

Goals for Today

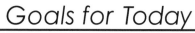

Gratitude Statement

• • • • • • • • • • • • •

Sleep the Night Before

• • • • • • • • • • • • • •

Celebrations & Struggles

• • • • • • • • • • • • •

DAILY JOURNAL

Date:

Food Journal

B

L

D

S

Habit Tracker

☆

☆

☆

☆

☆

☆

☆

Water Intake

Weight

Workout: Cardio Strength or Rest

Goals for Today

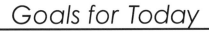

Gratitude Statement

Sleep the Night Before

Celebrations &Struggles

DAILY JOURNAL

Date: _____

Food Journal

B

L

D

S

Habit Tracker

☆
☆
☆
☆
☆
☆
☆

Water Intake

Weight

Workout: Cardio Strength or Rest

Goals for Today

Gratitude Statement

Sleep the Night Before

Celebrations & Struggles

DAILY JOURNAL

Date: _____

Food Journal

B

L

D

S

Habit Tracker

☆

☆

☆

☆

☆

☆

☆

Water Intake

Weight

•
•
•
•

Workout: Cardio Strength or Rest

• • • • • • • • • • • • • •

Goals for Today

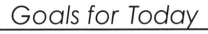

Gratitude Statement

• • • • • • • • • • • • • • •

Sleep the Night Before

• • • • • • • • • • • • • •

Celebrations & Struggles

• • • • • • • • • • • • • • •

DAILY JOURNAL

Date:

Food Journal

B

L

D

S

Habit Tracker

☆
☆
☆
☆
☆
☆
☆

Water Intake

Weight

Workout: Cardio Strength or Rest

Goals for Today

Gratitude Statement

Sleep the Night Before

Celebrations &Struggles

The Meal Planner

	BREAKFAST	LUNCH	DINNER	SNACKS
MON				
TUE				
WED				
THU				
FRI				
SAT				
SUN				

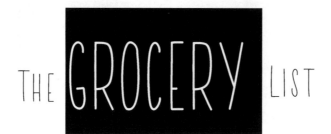

THE GROCERY LIST

Week Five:_____

DAILY JOURNAL

Date: _____

Food Journal

B

L

D

S

Habit Tracker

☆
☆
☆
☆
☆
☆
☆

Water Intake

Weight

Workout: Cardio Strength or Rest

Goals for Today

Gratitude Statement

Sleep the Night Before

Celebrations & Struggles

DAILY JOURNAL

Date: _____

Food Journal

B

L

D

S

Habit Tracker

☆
☆
☆
☆
☆
☆
☆

Water Intake

Weight

Workout: Cardio Strength or Rest

Goals for Today

Gratitude Statement

Sleep the Night Before

Celebrations & Struggles

DAILY JOURNAL

Date:_____

Food Journal

B

L

D

S

Habit Tracker

☆

☆

☆

☆

☆

☆

☆

Water Intake

Weight

Workout: Cardio Strength or Rest

Goals for Today

Gratitude Statement

Sleep the Night Before

Celebrations &Struggles

DAILY JOURNAL

Date:_____

Food Journal

B

L

D

S

Habit Tracker

☆
☆
☆
☆
☆
☆
☆

Water Intake

Weight

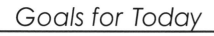

Workout: Cardio Strength or Rest

Goals for Today

Gratitude Statement

Sleep the Night Before

Celebrations & Struggles

DAILY JOURNAL

Date_____

Food Journal

B

L

D

S

Habit Tracker

☆

☆

☆

☆

☆

☆

☆

Water Intake

Weight

Workout: Cardio Strength or Rest

• • • • • • • • • • • • •

Goals for Today

Gratitude Statement

• • • • • • • • • • • •

Sleep the Night Before

• • • • • • • • • • •

Celebrations &Struggles

• • • • • • • • • • • •

DAILY JOURNAL

Date: _____

Food Journal

B

L

D

S

Habit Tracker

☆
☆
☆
☆
☆
☆
☆

Water Intake

Weight

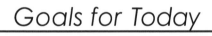

Workout: Cardio Strength or Rest

Goals for Today

Gratitude Statement

Sleep the Night Before

Celebrations & Struggles

DAILY JOURNAL

Date:

Food Journal

B

L

D

S

Habit Tracker

☆

☆

☆

☆

☆

☆

☆

Water Intake

Weight

Workout: Cardio Strength or Rest

Goals for Today

Gratitude Statement

Sleep the Night Before

Celebrations & Struggles

The Meal Planner

Week Six :

	BREAKFAST	LUNCH	DINNER	SNACKS
MON				
TUE				
WED				
THU				
FRI				
SAT				
SUN				

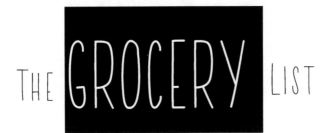

The GROCERY List

Week Six:_____

- □ _____
- □ _____
- □ _____
- □ _____
- □ _____
- □ _____
- □ _____
- □ _____
- □ _____

- □ _____
- □ _____
- □ _____
- □ _____
- □ _____
- □ _____
- □ _____
- □ _____
- □ _____

- □ _____
- □ _____
- □ _____
- □ _____
- □ _____
- □ _____
- □ _____
- □ _____
- □ _____

- □ _____
- □ _____
- □ _____
- □ _____
- □ _____
- □ _____
- □ _____
- □ _____
- □ _____

DAILY JOURNAL

Date:_____

Food Journal

B

L

D

S

Habit Tracker

☆
☆
☆
☆
☆
☆
☆

Water Intake

Weight

Workout: Cardio Strength or Rest

Goals for Today

Gratitude Statement

Sleep the Night Before

Celebrations & Struggles

DAILY JOURNAL

Date: _____

Food Journal

B

L

D

S

Habit Tracker

☆
☆
☆
☆
☆
☆
☆

Water Intake

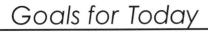

Weight

Workout: Cardio Strength or Rest

• • • • • • • • • • • • • • • •

Goals for Today

Gratitude Statement

• • • • • • • • • • • • • •

Sleep the Night Before

• • • • • • • • • • • • • • •

Celebrations & Struggles

• • • • • • • • • • • • • • • •

DAILY JOURNAL

Date:_____

Food Journal

B

L

D

S

Habit Tracker

☆

☆

☆

☆

☆

☆

☆

Water Intake

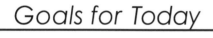

Weight

Workout: Cardio Strength or Rest

• • • • • • • • • • • • • • • • •

Goals for Today

Gratitude Statement

• • • • • • • • • • • • • • • •

Sleep the Night Before

• • • • • • • • • • • • • • • •

Celebrations &Struggles

• • • • • • • • • • • • • • • •

DAILY JOURNAL

Date: _____

Food Journal

B

L

D

S

Habit Tracker

☆

☆

☆

☆

☆

☆

☆

Water Intake

Weight

Workout: Cardio Strength or Rest

• • • • • • • • • • • • • •

Goals for Today

Gratitude Statement

• • • • • • • • • • • • •

Sleep the Night Before

• • • • • • • • • • • • •

Celebrations & Struggles

• • • • • • • • • • • • •

DAILY JOURNAL

Date: _____

Food Journal

B

L

D

S

Habit Tracker

☆

☆

☆

☆

☆

☆

☆

Water Intake

Weight

Workout: Cardio Strength or Rest

Goals for Today

Gratitude Statement

Sleep the Night Before

Celebrations & Struggles

DAILY JOURNAL

Date:

Food Journal

B

L

D

S

Habit Tracker

☆

☆

☆

☆

☆

☆

☆

Water Intake

Weight

Workout: Cardio Strength or Rest

Goals for Today

Gratitude Statement

Sleep the Night Before

Celebrations & Struggles

DAILY JOURNAL

Date: _____

Food Journal

B

L

D

S

Habit Tracker

☆

☆

☆

☆

☆

☆

☆

Water Intake

Weight

Workout: Cardio Strength or Rest

Goals for Today

Gratitude Statement

Sleep the Night Before

Celebrations & Struggles

The Meal Planner

	BREAKFAST	LUNCH	DINNER	SNACKS
MON				
TUE				
WED				
THU				
FRI				
SAT				
SUN				

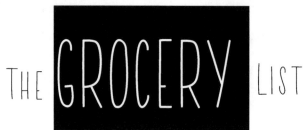

THE GROCERY LIST

Week Seven:_____

DAILY JOURNAL

Date _____

Food Journal

B

L

D

S

Habit Tracker

☆
☆
☆
☆
☆
☆
☆

Water Intake

Weight

Workout: Cardio Strength or Rest

Goals for Today

Gratitude Statement

Sleep the Night Before

Celebrations & Struggles

DAILY JOURNAL

Date _____

Food Journal

B

L

D

S

Habit Tracker

☆
☆
☆
☆
☆
☆
☆

Water Intake

Weight

Workout: Cardio Strength or Rest

Goals for Today

Gratitude Statement

Sleep the Night Before

Celebrations &Struggles

DAILY JOURNAL

Date: _____

Food Journal

B

L

D

S

Habit Tracker

☆

☆

☆

☆

☆

☆

☆

Water Intake

Weight

Workout: Cardio Strength or Rest

Goals for Today

Gratitude Statement

Sleep the Night Before

Celebrations &Struggles

DAILY JOURNAL

Food Journal

B

L

D

S

Habit Tracker

☆

☆

☆

☆

☆

☆

☆

Water Intake

Weight

Workout: Cardio Strength or Rest

Goals for Today

Gratitude Statement

Sleep the Night Before

Celebrations &Struggles

DAILY JOURNAL

Date: _____

Food Journal

B

L

D

S

Habit Tracker

☆

☆

☆

☆

☆

☆

☆

Water Intake

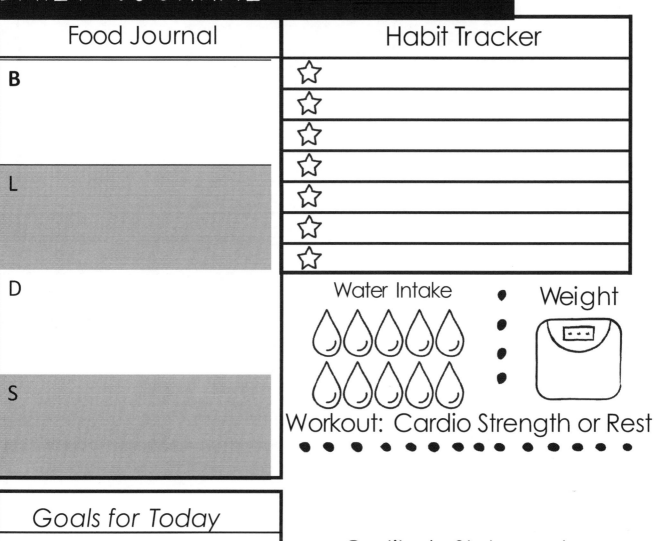

Weight

Workout: Cardio Strength or Rest

Goals for Today

Gratitude Statement

Sleep the Night Before

Celebrations &Struggles

DAILY JOURNAL

Date_____

Food Journal

B

L

D

S

Habit Tracker

☆
☆
☆
☆
☆
☆
☆

Water Intake

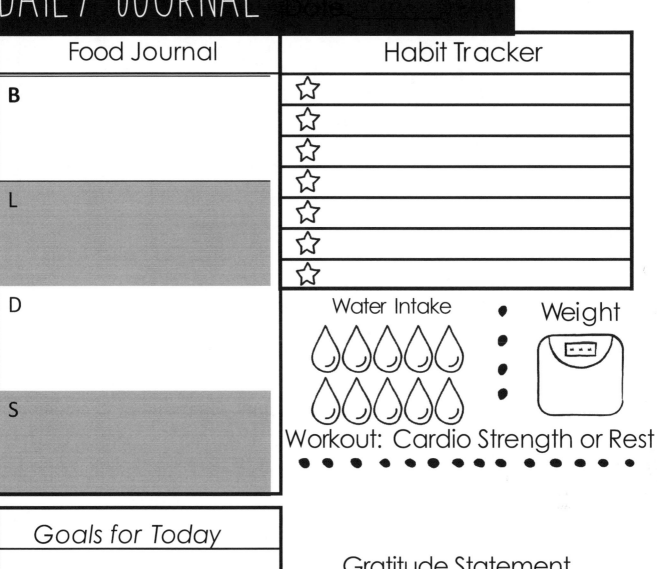

Weight

Workout: Cardio Strength or Rest

Goals for Today

Gratitude Statement

Sleep the Night Before

Celebrations & Struggles

DAILY JOURNAL

Date _____

Food Journal

B

L

D

S

Habit Tracker

☆

☆

☆

☆

☆

☆

☆

Water Intake

Weight

Workout: Cardio Strength or Rest

Goals for Today

Gratitude Statement

Sleep the Night Before

Celebrations &Struggles

The Meal Planner

	BREAKFAST	LUNCH	DINNER	SNACKS
MON				
TUE				
WED				
THU				
FRI				
SAT				
SUN				

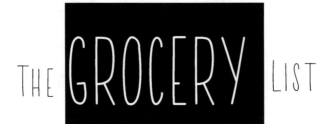

The GROCERY List

Week Eight:_____

DAILY JOURNAL

Date

Food Journal

B

L

D

S

Habit Tracker

☆

☆

☆

☆

☆

☆

☆

Water Intake

Weight

Workout: Cardio Strength or Rest

Goals for Today

Gratitude Statement

Sleep the Night Before

Celebrations & Struggles

DAILY JOURNAL

Date: _____

Food Journal

B

L

D

S

Habit Tracker

☆

☆

☆

☆

☆

☆

☆

Water Intake

Weight

Workout: Cardio Strength or Rest
• • • • • • • • • • • • • • •

Goals for Today

Gratitude Statement
• • • • • • • • • • • • •

Sleep the Night Before
• • • • • • • • • • • • • •

Celebrations & Struggles
• • • • • • • • • • • • • •

DAILY JOURNAL

Food Journal

B

L

D

S

Habit Tracker

☆

☆

☆

☆

☆

☆

☆

Water Intake

Weight

Workout: Cardio Strength or Rest

Goals for Today

Gratitude Statement

Sleep the Night Before

Celebrations & Struggles

DAILY JOURNAL

Date: _____

Food Journal

B

L

D

S

Habit Tracker

☆

☆

☆

☆

☆

☆

☆

Water Intake

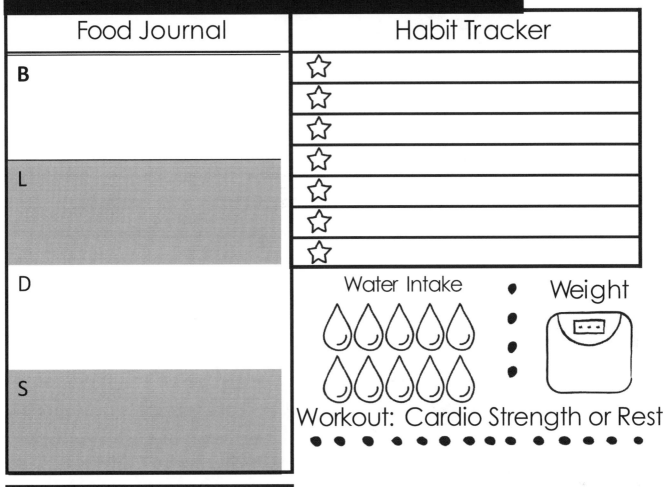

Weight

Workout: Cardio Strength or Rest

• • • • • • • • • • • • • • • • • •

Goals for Today

Gratitude Statement

• • • • • • • • • • • • • • • •

Sleep the Night Before

• • • • • • • • • • • • • • • •

Celebrations & Struggles

• • • • • • • • • • • • • • • •

DAILY JOURNAL

Date

Food Journal

B

L

D

S

Habit Tracker

☆

☆

☆

☆

☆

☆

☆

Water Intake

Weight

Workout: Cardio Strength or Rest

● ● ● ● ● ● ● ● ● ● ● ● ● ●

Goals for Today

Gratitude Statement

Sleep the Night Before

Celebrations &Struggles

DAILY JOURNAL

Date: _____

Food Journal

B

L

D

S

Habit Tracker

☆

☆

☆

☆

☆

☆

☆

Water Intake

Weight

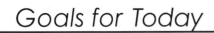

Workout: Cardio Strength or Rest

Goals for Today

Gratitude Statement

Sleep the Night Before

Celebrations &Struggles

DAILY JOURNAL

Date:

Food Journal

B

L

D

S

Habit Tracker

☆
☆
☆
☆
☆
☆
☆

Water Intake

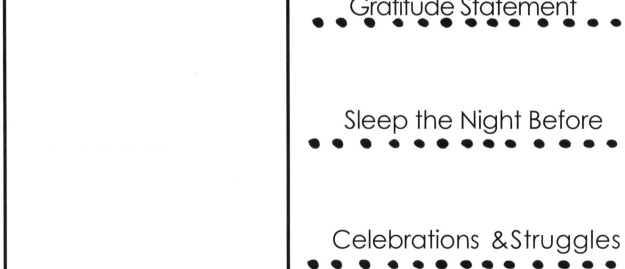

Weight

Workout: Cardio Strength or Rest

Goals for Today

Gratitude Statement

Sleep the Night Before

Celebrations &Struggles

The Meal Planner

	BREAKFAST	LUNCH	DINNER	SNACKS
MON				
TUE				
WED				
THU				
FRI				
SAT				
SUN				

The GROCERY List

DAILY JOURNAL

Date: _____

Food Journal

B

L

D

S

Habit Tracker

☆

☆

☆

☆

☆

☆

☆

Water Intake

Weight

Workout: Cardio Strength or Rest

Goals for Today

Gratitude Statement

Sleep the Night Before

Celebrations & Struggles

DAILY JOURNAL

Date

Food Journal

B

L

D

S

Habit Tracker

☆

☆

☆

☆

☆

☆

☆

Water Intake

Weight

Workout: Cardio Strength or Rest

• • • • • • • • • • • • • • • • • •

Goals for Today

Gratitude Statement

• • • • • • • • • • • • • • • • • •

Sleep the Night Before

• • • • • • • • • • • • • • • • • •

Celebrations &Struggles

• • • • • • • • • • • • • • • • • •

DAILY JOURNAL

Date: _____

Food Journal

B

L

D

S

Habit Tracker

☆
☆
☆
☆
☆
☆
☆

Water Intake

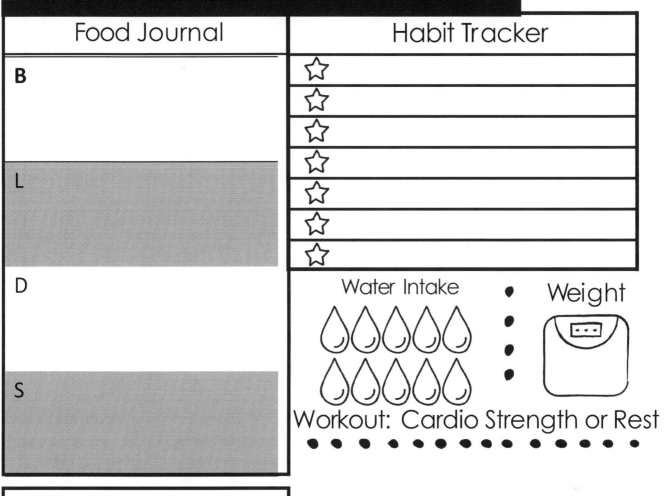

Weight

Workout: Cardio Strength or Rest

Goals for Today

Gratitude Statement

Sleep the Night Before

Celebrations & Struggles

DAILY JOURNAL

Date:

Food Journal

B

L

D

S

Habit Tracker

☆

☆

☆

☆

☆

☆

☆

Water Intake

Weight

Workout: Cardio Strength or Rest

Goals for Today

Gratitude Statement

Sleep the Night Before

Celebrations & Struggles

DAILY JOURNAL

Date:_____

Food Journal

B

L

D

S

Habit Tracker

☆

☆

☆

☆

☆

☆

☆

Water Intake

Weight

Workout: Cardio Strength or Rest

Goals for Today

Gratitude Statement

Sleep the Night Before

Celebrations &Struggles

DAILY JOURNAL

Date: _____

Food Journal

B

L

D

S

Habit Tracker

☆

☆

☆

☆

☆

☆

☆

Water Intake

Weight

Workout: Cardio Strength or Rest

Goals for Today

Gratitude Statement

Sleep the Night Before

Celebrations & Struggles

DAILY JOURNAL

Date: _____

Food Journal

B

L

D

S

Habit Tracker

☆
☆
☆
☆
☆
☆
☆

Water Intake

Weight

Workout: Cardio Strength or Rest

Goals for Today

Gratitude Statement

Sleep the Night Before

Celebrations &Struggles

The Meal Planner

	BREAKFAST	LUNCH	DINNER	SNACKS
MON				
TUE				
WED				
THU				
FRI				
SAT				
SUN				

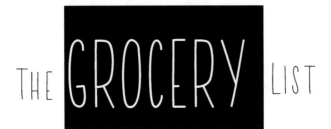

The GROCERY List

Week Ten:_____

DAILY JOURNAL

Date:

Food Journal

B

L

D

S

Habit Tracker

☆

☆

☆

☆

☆

☆

☆

Water Intake

Weight

Workout: Cardio Strength or Rest

Goals for Today

Gratitude Statement

Sleep the Night Before

Celebrations & Struggles

DAILY JOURNAL

Date: _____

Food Journal

B

L

D

S

Habit Tracker

☆

☆

☆

☆

☆

☆

☆

Water Intake

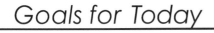

Weight

Workout: Cardio Strength or Rest

Goals for Today

Gratitude Statement

Sleep the Night Before

Celebrations & Struggles

DAILY JOURNAL

Date:

Food Journal

B

L

D

S

Habit Tracker

☆

☆

☆

☆

☆

☆

☆

Water Intake

Weight

Workout: Cardio Strength or Rest

Goals for Today

Gratitude Statement

Sleep the Night Before

Celebrations & Struggles

DAILY JOURNAL

Date:_____

Food Journal

B

L

D

S

Habit Tracker

☆
☆
☆
☆
☆
☆
☆

Water Intake

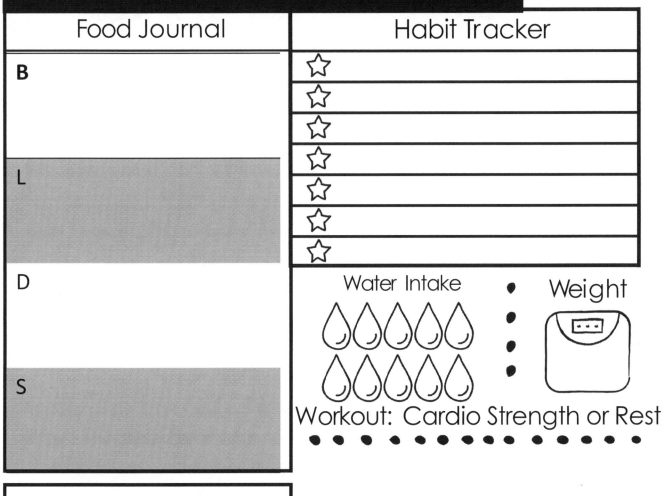

Weight

Workout: Cardio Strength or Rest

Goals for Today

Gratitude Statement

Sleep the Night Before

Celebrations &Struggles

DAILY JOURNAL

Date

Food Journal

B

L

D

S

Habit Tracker

☆

☆

☆

☆

☆

☆

☆

Water Intake

Weight

Workout: Cardio Strength or Rest

Goals for Today

Gratitude Statement

Sleep the Night Before

Celebrations &Struggles

DAILY JOURNAL

Date:_____

Food Journal

B

L

D

S

Habit Tracker

☆

☆

☆

☆

☆

☆

☆

Water Intake

Weight

Workout: Cardio Strength or Rest

Goals for Today

Gratitude Statement

Sleep the Night Before

Celebrations &Struggles

DAILY JOURNAL

Date:

Food Journal

B

L

D

S

Habit Tracker

☆
☆
☆
☆
☆
☆
☆

Water Intake

Weight

Workout: Cardio Strength or Rest

Goals for Today

Gratitude Statement

Sleep the Night Before

Celebrations & Struggles

The Meal Planner

	BREAKFAST	LUNCH	DINNER	SNACKS
MON				
TUE				
WED				
THU				
FRI				
SAT				
SUN				

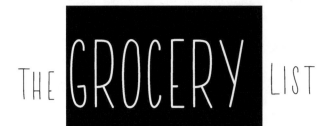

The GROCERY List

Week Eleven:_____

DAILY JOURNAL

Date:

Food Journal

B

L

D

S

Habit Tracker

☆
☆
☆
☆
☆
☆
☆

Water Intake

Weight

Workout: Cardio Strength or Rest

Goals for Today

Gratitude Statement

Sleep the Night Before

Celebrations &Struggles

DAILY JOURNAL

Date

Food Journal

B

L

D

S

Habit Tracker

☆

☆

☆

☆

☆

☆

☆

Water Intake

Weight

Workout: Cardio Strength or Rest

Goals for Today

Gratitude Statement

Sleep the Night Before

Celebrations & Struggles

DAILY JOURNAL

Date: _____

Food Journal

B

L

D

S

Habit Tracker

☆

☆

☆

☆

☆

☆

☆

Water Intake

Weight

Workout: Cardio Strength or Rest

Goals for Today

Gratitude Statement

Sleep the Night Before

Celebrations &Struggles

DAILY JOURNAL

Date:

Food Journal

B

L

D

S

Habit Tracker

☆
☆
☆
☆
☆
☆
☆

Water Intake

Weight

Workout: Cardio Strength or Rest

Goals for Today

Gratitude Statement

Sleep the Night Before

Celebrations & Struggles

DAILY JOURNAL

Date:_____

Food Journal

B

L

D

S

Habit Tracker

☆

☆

☆

☆

☆

☆

☆

Water Intake

Weight

Workout: Cardio Strength or Rest

Goals for Today

Gratitude Statement

Sleep the Night Before

Celebrations &Struggles

DAILY JOURNAL

Date _____

Food Journal

B

L

D

S

Habit Tracker

☆
☆
☆
☆
☆
☆
☆

Water Intake

Weight

Workout: Cardio Strength or Rest

Goals for Today

Gratitude Statement

Sleep the Night Before

Celebrations & Struggles

DAILY JOURNAL

Date: _____

Food Journal

B

L

D

S

Habit Tracker

☆
☆
☆
☆
☆
☆
☆

Water Intake

Weight

Workout: Cardio Strength or Rest

Goals for Today

Gratitude Statement

Sleep the Night Before

Celebrations & Struggles

The Meal Planner

	BREAKFAST	LUNCH	DINNER	SNACKS
MON				
TUE				
WED				
THU				
FRI				
SAT				
SUN				

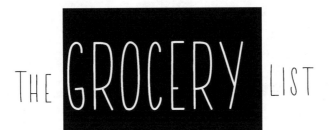

The GROCERY List

Week Twelve:_____

DAILY JOURNAL

Date _____

Food Journal

B

L

D

S

Habit Tracker

☆

☆

☆

☆

☆

☆

☆

Water Intake

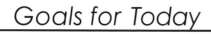

Weight

Workout: Cardio Strength or Rest
● ● ● ● ● ● ● ● ● ● ● ● ● ● ● ●

Goals for Today

Gratitude Statement
● ● ● ● ● ● ● ● ● ● ● ● ● ●

Sleep the Night Before
● ● ● ● ● ● ● ● ● ● ● ● ● ●

Celebrations & Struggles
● ● ● ● ● ● ● ● ● ● ● ● ● ● ●

DAILY JOURNAL

Date: _____

Food Journal

B

L

D

S

Habit Tracker

☆

☆

☆

☆

☆

☆

☆

Water Intake

Weight

Workout: Cardio Strength or Rest

Goals for Today

Gratitude Statement

Sleep the Night Before

Celebrations &Struggles

DAILY JOURNAL

Food Journal

B

L

D

S

Habit Tracker

☆

☆

☆

☆

☆

☆

☆

Water Intake

Weight

Workout: Cardio Strength or Rest

Goals for Today

Gratitude Statement

Sleep the Night Before

Celebrations &Struggles

DAILY JOURNAL

Date:_____

Food Journal

B

L

D

S

Habit Tracker

☆

☆

☆

☆

☆

☆

☆

Water Intake

Weight

Workout: Cardio Strength or Rest

• • • • • • • • • • • • • • • • •

Goals for Today

Gratitude Statement

• • • • • • • • • • • • • • •

Sleep the Night Before

• • • • • • • • • • • • • • •

Celebrations &Struggles

• • • • • • • • • • • • • • •

DAILY JOURNAL

Date: _____

Food Journal

B

L

D

S

Habit Tracker

☆
☆
☆
☆
☆
☆
☆

Water Intake

Weight

Workout: Cardio Strength or Rest

Goals for Today

Gratitude Statement

Sleep the Night Before

Celebrations & Struggles

DAILY JOURNAL

Date:_____

Food Journal

B

L

D

S

Habit Tracker

☆

☆

☆

☆

☆

☆

☆

Water Intake

Weight

Workout: Cardio Strength or Rest

• • • • • • • • • • • • • • •

Goals for Today

Gratitude Statement

• • • • • • • • • • • • • • •

Sleep the Night Before

• • • • • • • • • • • • • • •

Celebrations &Struggles

• • • • • • • • • • • • • • •

DAILY JOURNAL

Date: _____

Food Journal

B

L

D

S

Habit Tracker

☆

☆

☆

☆

☆

☆

☆

Water Intake

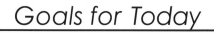

Weight

● ● ● ●

Workout: Cardio Strength or Rest

● ● ● ● ● ● ● ● ● ● ● ● ● ●

Goals for Today

Gratitude Statement

● ● ● ● ● ● ● ● ● ● ● ● ● ● ● ● ●

Sleep the Night Before

● ● ● ● ● ● ● ● ● ● ● ●

Celebrations & Struggles

● ● ● ● ● ● ● ● ● ● ● ● ● ●

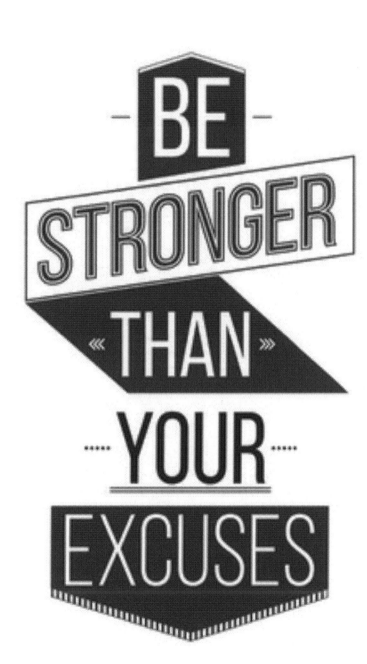

BE STRONGER THAN YOUR EXCUSES

WORKOUT SCHEDULE

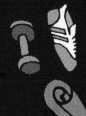

JAN FEB MAR APR MAY JUN JUL AUG SEPT OCT NOV DEC

	Sunday	Monday	Tuesday	Wednesday	Thursday	Friday	Saturday
	Cardio Strength Rest	Cardio Strength Rest	Cardio Strength Rest	Cardio Strength Rest	Cardio Strength Rest	Cardio Strength Rest	Cardio Strength Rest
	Cardio Strength Rest	Cardio Strength Rest	Cardio Strength Rest	Cardio Strength Rest	Cardio Strength Rest	Cardio Strength Rest	Cardio Strength Rest
	Cardio Strength Rest	Cardio Strength Rest	Cardio Strength Rest	Cardio Strength Rest	Cardio Strength Rest	Cardio Strength Rest	Cardio Strength Rest
	Cardio Strength Rest	Cardio Strength Rest	Cardio Strength Rest	Cardio Strength Rest	Cardio Strength Rest	Cardio Strength Rest	Cardio Strength Rest
	Cardio Strength Rest	Cardio Strength Rest	Cardio Strength Rest	Cardio Strength Rest	Cardio Strength Rest	Cardio Strength Rest	Cardio Strength Rest

WORKOUT SCHEDULE

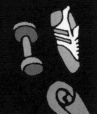

JAN FEB MAR APR MAY
JUN JUL AUG SEPT OCT
NOV DEC

	Sunday	Monday	Tuesday	Wednesday	Thursday	Friday	Saturday
	Cardio Strength Rest	Cardio Strength Rest	Cardio Strength Rest	Cardio Strength Rest	Cardio Strength Rest	Cardio Strength Rest	Cardio Strength Rest
	Cardio Strength Rest	Cardio Strength Rest	Cardio Strength Rest	Cardio Strength Rest	Cardio Strength Rest	Cardio Strength Rest	Cardio Strength Rest
	Cardio Strength Rest	Cardio Strength Rest	Cardio Strength Rest	Cardio Strength Rest	Cardio Strength Rest	Cardio Strength Rest	Cardio Strength Rest
	Cardio Strength Rest	Cardio Strength Rest	Cardio Strength Rest	Cardio Strength Rest	Cardio Strength Rest	Cardio Strength Rest	Cardio Strength Rest
		Cardio Strength Rest	Cardio Strength Rest	Cardio Strength Rest	Cardio Strength Rest	Cardio Strength Rest	Cardio Strength Rest

WORKOUT SCHEDULE

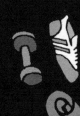

JAN FEB MAR APR MAY
JUN JUL AUG SEPT OCT
NOV DEC

	Sunday	Monday	Tuesday	Wednesday	Thursday	Friday	Saturday
	Cardio Strength Rest	Cardio Strength Rest	Cardio Strength Rest	Cardio Strength Rest	Cardio Strength Rest	Cardio Strength Rest	Cardio Strength Rest
	Cardio Strength Rest	Cardio Strength Rest	Cardio Strength Rest	Cardio Strength Rest	Cardio Strength Rest	Cardio Strength Rest	Cardio Strength Rest
	Cardio Strength Rest	Cardio Strength Rest	Cardio Strength Rest	Cardio Strength Rest	Cardio Strength Rest	Cardio Strength Rest	Cardio Strength Rest
	Cardio Strength Rest	Cardio Strength Rest	Cardio Strength Rest	Cardio Strength Rest	Cardio Strength Rest	Cardio Strength Rest	Cardio Strength Rest
	Cardio Strength Rest	Cardio Strength Rest	Cardio Strength Rest	Cardio Strength Rest	Cardio Strength Rest	Cardio Strength Rest	Cardio Strength Rest

CARDIO CHECK IN MONTH 1

Date	Activity	Time	Distance	Calories	Rating
					☆☆☆
					☆☆☆
					☆☆☆
					☆☆☆
					☆☆☆
					☆☆☆
					☆☆☆
					☆☆☆
					☆☆☆
					☆☆☆
					☆☆☆
					☆☆☆
					☆☆☆
					☆☆☆
					☆☆☆
					☆☆☆
					☆☆☆
					☆☆☆
					☆☆☆
					☆☆☆
					☆☆☆

CARDIO CHECK IN MONTH 2

Date	Activity	Time	Distance	Calories	Rating
					☆☆☆
					☆☆☆
					☆☆☆
					☆☆☆
					☆☆☆
					☆☆☆
					☆☆☆
					☆☆☆
					☆☆☆
					☆☆☆
					☆☆☆
					☆☆☆
					☆☆☆
					☆☆☆
					☆☆☆
					☆☆☆
					☆☆☆
					☆☆☆
					☆☆☆
					☆☆☆
					☆☆☆
					☆☆☆

CARDIO CHECK IN MONTH 3

Date	Activity	Time	Distance	Calories	Rating
					☆☆☆
					☆☆☆
					☆☆☆
					☆☆☆
					☆☆☆
					☆☆☆
					☆☆☆
					☆☆☆
					☆☆☆
					☆☆☆
					☆☆☆
					☆☆☆
					☆☆☆
					☆☆☆
					☆☆☆
					☆☆☆
					☆☆☆
					☆☆☆
					☆☆☆
					☆☆☆
					☆☆☆

Strength training Week 1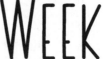

	description	weight	sets	Reps	Notes

	description	weight	sets	Reps	Notes

	description	weight	sets	Reps	Notes

Strength training Week 2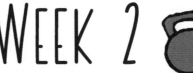

	description	weight	sets	Reps	Notes

	description	weight	sets	Reps	Notes

	description	weight	sets	Reps	Notes

Strength training   Week 3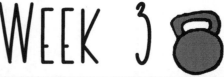

description	weight	sets	Reps	Notes

description	weight	sets	Reps	Notes

description	weight	sets	Reps	Notes

Strength training Week 4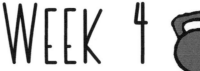

	description	weight	sets	Reps	Notes

	description	weight	sets	Reps	Notes

	description	weight	sets	Reps	Notes

Strength training Week 5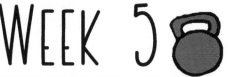

	description	weight	sets	Reps	Notes

	description	weight	sets	Reps	Notes

	description	weight	sets	Reps	Notes

Strength Training Week 6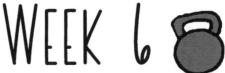

	description	weight	sets	Reps	Notes

	description	weight	sets	Reps	Notes

	description	weight	sets	Reps	Notes

STRENGTH TRAINING Week 7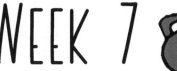

	description	weight	sets	Reps	Notes

	description	weight	sets	Reps	Notes

	description	weight	sets	Reps	Notes

Strength training Week 8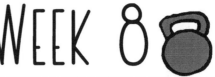

	description	weight	sets	Reps	Notes

	description	weight	sets	Reps	Notes

	description	weight	sets	Reps	Notes

Strength training Week 9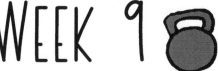

description	weight	sets	Reps	Notes

description	weight	sets	Reps	Notes

description	weight	sets	Reps	Notes

Strength training Week 10

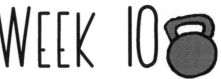

description	weight	sets	Reps	Notes

description	weight	sets	Reps	Notes

description	weight	sets	Reps	Notes

Strength training Week 11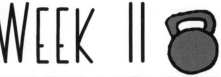

description	weight	sets	Reps	Notes

description	weight	sets	Reps	Notes

description	weight	sets	Reps	Notes

Strength training   Week 12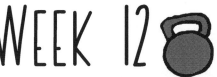

description	weight	sets	Reps	Notes

description	weight	sets	Reps	Notes

description	weight	sets	Reps	Notes

Made in United States
Troutdale, OR
10/09/2023

13543316R00080